YOUR GUIDE TO A
SAFE AND SWIFT
HOSPITAL STAY

YOUR GUIDE TO A SAFE AND SWIFT HOSPITAL STAY

by

Maureen Healy, MSN, APRN

Family Nurse Practitioner
Healthcare Educator & Advocate

Based on a True Story

Your Guide to a Safe and Swift Hospital Stay
by Maureen Healy, MSN, APRN
Family Nurse Practitioner
Healthcare Educator & Advocate

ISBN: 978-1-7334074-0-3
Library of Congress Control Number: 2020931922

Published in the United States of America

While the author made every effort to provide accurate information at the time of publication, neither the publisher nor the author assumes any responsibility for errors, or for changes that may occur after publication.

This handbook is not intended as a substitute for the medical advice of physicians. The reader should regularly consult a physician in matters relating to his/her health and particularly with respect to any symptoms that may require diagnosis or medical attention.

Dedication

This book is dedicated to my mom, Mary C. Healy,
her two sisters, Kathleen O'Donnell and Carolyn D. Bennett,
and to my cousin, Margie O'Donnell Schuchts.

These women were registered nurses. They instilled invaluable
knowledge in those they touched and were deeply loved by those
they knew.

And for my dad,
Raymond W. Healy, MD
who, in 1953, was the first general practitioner
in North Miami Beach, Florida.

His practice of medicine was far ahead of his time.
He started me on my nursing journey when I was 14.

May they all rest in peace.

Contents

Preface

URING MY FIRST MONTH working as a brand new reg- istered nurse, the nurse manager taped a newspaper article in the medicine room, so it was visible to the staff. The headline read, "Drug Errors Do KILL." It talked about a common potassium medication, one that would not harm 99% of us. However, in this case, the drug was given to a patient in kidney failure who had a long history of renal disease. It killed her.

As I acknowledged the horrible consequences asso- ciated with giving someone the wrong medication, the reality of my new profession set in. Profoundly affected, I told myself to slow down, follow protocols, and observe hospital guidelines. That incident also reinforced that I wanted to go through my career never harming anyone. Over thirty years later, so far, so good!

Fifteen years after that eye-opening experience, I was working in the Emergency department when my mom was involved in a near-fatal motor vehicle accident. Be- cause she was in her seventies, she was at greater risk for potential complications. These preventable complications included pneumonia, infection, and blood clots. The danger period starts within 48 hours of being hospitalized, and it can last well after being discharged home. I wanted Mom's recovery to be uneventful and speedy, as I was determined she would not deteriorate on my watch. As a result, I used all the nursing knowledge I had acquired over the years and applied them on a daily basis. It took her four months to fully recover—without any setbacks!

The following summer at our family reunion, I was reliving the experience. It was my cousin Margie and her sister Ann, another registered nurse, who made me realize the positive outcome was because of what I did during my mom's recovery. I recall saying all I did was insist she got up out of bed (no matter how much it hurt), brought in better food choices, and made her laugh or, at least smile. I can still hear Margie saying, "Yes Mimi, that's what you did. You made her get out of bed and walk, you gave her foods that helped her heal. You encouraged smiling so she felt better. That got her through the ordeal without any complications. No infections, no blood clots, no pneumonia."

When I returned to work, it seemed many of my patients' families were asking what they should do to help. That's when the light bulb went off in my head, and this book was conceived. I began passionately teaching all of my patients, their families, and friends tips to prevent complications, errors, and mishaps, while promoting a speedy hospital recovery.

I believe the modern method of patient advocacy embraces a trilateral support structure where every aspect of care is managed by separate, yet unified entities to act in the best interests of the patients. That triangle is comprised of doctors, nurses, and family members (including friends and caregivers).

This handbook's **PAINFREE** approach teaches families and caregivers how to get involved and stay involved in a positive collaboration for a positive outcome. The acronym is used as an easy reference that covers all the steps for achieving the goal of an uneventful hospital recovery.

"P" Patient Advocate
"A" Ambulate
"I" Infection
"N" Nutrition
"F" Faith
"R" Remember to Follow-up
"E" Eliminate
"E" Educate

Why Be a Part of the HealthCare Team?

When patients are admitted into the hospital, they become the "quarterback." The quarterback is the most valuable player. Every other position is designed to help the quarterback succeed. On the front lines are the doctors and nurses. The skilled positions (wide receivers and running backs) are there to help the quarterback make progress by moving the ball down the field—towards recovery. These are the people in the pharmacy, radiology, lab, and respiratory departments, as well as the physical/occupational therapists, the nutritionists, and all the other members of the team.

However, the players are not the most important part of a football team. The coaches are the most important. Families, friends, and caregivers become instant coaches when their loved one is hospitalized. The coaches are active participants in the game. They watch the plays, observing who is doing what, making sure all team players are working well together (jobs are getting done as ordered), intervene when necessary, and make their voices heard when something is wrong.

This guide aims to be the playbook for the coaches so they can steer their quarterback home safely.

By imparting knowledge to families and caregivers about their participation as active members of the healthcare team, we will improve the lives of all patients to come.

It is my hope that universities will add this triangular model into their School of Nursing curriculums, that all nursing students will learn to incorporate this system into their nursing practice, and that the world's largest healthcare organizations will promote the value of its concepts.

Introduction

I T IS A SCARY EVENT when an unexpected accident or serious illness causes a trip to the hospital. Once inside the hospital, you become part of the hectic atmosphere. Most of us are overwhelmed by these unfamiliar sounds, smells, and sights. However, you want to keep a clear head to help your loved one stay calm. Actively participating in all aspects of the patient's care will promote a safe recovery and swift discharge home.

Hospitals are stressful environments. They create opportunities for distractions and unforeseen healthcare errors. Studies show that in U.S. hospitals, 250,000 people die annually from preventable errors.[1] The exact number is difficult to calculate because there are many variables to take into account. Errors are defined as any mistake while receiving medical care and includes medicines, surgery, diagnoses, labs and other test results.[2]

There are also several "nursing factors" that play a role in these preventable errors. First, there is the nursing shortage issue. Second, there are the frequent interruptions that occur while nurses are preparing and administering medications. Another factor is when patients stay in bed for extended periods of time. Prolonged bedrest leads to more health complications and an overall worsening of their condition. These potential circumstantial errors can lead to longer hospital stays, increased personal stress, and expense.

Survey findings from various healthcare affiliates reveal key data about nurses in the workforce today and what the future holds for them.

According to the Bureau of Labor Statistics' Employment Projections for 2016-2026, the registered nurses' workforce is expected to grow from 2.9 million in 2016 to 3.4 million in 2026 which is a 15% increase.[3]

However, in July 2017, the *Journal of Nursing Regulation* documented research that projects 1 million RNs will *retire* by 2030.[4] This equates to 1.5 million job vacancies for registered nurses over the next decade! This substantial loss will affect patient care and ultimately, patient outcome.[5]

The Agency for Healthcare Research and Quality (AHRQ) published a meta-analysis in 2007 that simply stated, "with inadequate staffing, patient safety is compromised."[6]

Nursing schools are turning away thousands of qualified applicants according to the American Association of College of Nursing (AACN) "due to the insufficient number of faculty, clinical sites, classroom space, and clinical preceptors, as well as budget constraints." The main contributing factor to fewer students is reflected by the number of faculty members retiring. The faculty members along with the RN workforce are on average, over age 50. If fewer nurses are graduating, fewer are at the bedside. This lack of bedside nursing directly compromises patient outcomes and most likely will increase patient mortality.[7]

To make matters worse, there's the aging population! The U.S. Census Bureau, in May 2014, stated that more than 20% of the U.S. population will be over 65 years of age by 2030.[8] Besides the obvious increase in caring for chronic conditions, there will be a continued rise of debilitating health issues associated with Alzheimer's and dementia-related diseases.[9]

Now let's go back into the hospital for an understanding of the hospital flow.

On any medical floor, the reality of doctors' and nurses' roles—what is truly taking place to care for *one patient* on any given day—looks like this in today's world.

The admitting physician, specialty physicians, and surgeons (i.e., Cardiac, Pulmonary, Orthopedic, etc.), and their nurse practitioners/physician assistants diagnose and treat each patient, generating a multitude of orders to be managed by *an individual* RN which includes:

More medications,
More tests,
More procedures,
More blood work,
More IVs,
More equipment.

All of these tasks require detailed computer documentation on sicker patients who tend to have multiple chronic conditions. In addition, there is the extra time and challenge spent communicating with patients who present with language barriers.

This barely highlights the many responsibilities one Registered Nurse (RN) has with one patient. He/she can have five to ten patients depending on the hospital floor. Each physician works up the patient based on their expertise in regard to the patient's problem(s). The more comorbidities (multiple chronic conditions, for example, hypertension, diabetes, and/or heart disease), the greater the number of physicians who will get involved. It is not unusual to have three or four different doctors plus their nurse practitioners and physician assistants doing rounds on any given patient.

The RN must confirm all the orders are implemented, and then follow-up with all the results. If there are any abnormal results, it is top priority to notify the ordering physician who will most likely order more tests or treatments to address the abnormality.

This goes beyond all the general nursing duties an RN has for each patient: administering medications on time, taking vital signs, testing blood sugars, delivering pain control, and all the necessary tasks for helping the sick and their families; including those unforeseen issues that arise requiring immediate assistance.

Unforeseen issues include equipment not working or not available, bleeding, vomiting, diarrhea, or countless other unexpected problems demanding the RN to stop, change focus to deal with the most urgent issue, then return to the current jobs also requiring immediate attention. Meanwhile, there is ALWAYS the continued watch and awareness for patient safety.

As you can see, time is a luxury nurses don't have. And it's not just nurses who are in a hurry and may feel stressed. It's everyone involved, from physicians and pharmacists, to the inter-departments (Lab, Radiology, Dietary, Environmental Services); essentially, the entire hospital staff.

Families and friends are under tremendous stress as well. They're visiting a rapid-paced environment full of unfamiliar faces. They're often bewildered by the terminology and the tests. The nurse is therefore also kept busy keeping everyone informed of the current situation.

With all the knowledge, computers, and technology available to help mitigate a mishap, nothing can replace the power of touch or the value of an extra pair of eyes to watch over the patient. A familiar voice offering words of encouragement also goes a long way to enhance a patient's overall recovery.

This is where families and caregivers become part of the healthcare team. The RN is the link between all the healthcare team players. It is the RN's job to make sure the quarterback gets everything he/she needs in order to return home.

The Affordable Care Act "puts consumers back in charge of their healthcare." Under the law, a new Patient's Bill of Rights gives the American people the stability and flexibility they need to make informed choices about their health.[10]

This book is designed to take "informed choices" one step further. The reader will gain a proactive perspective of what to think about and what can be done to ensure a safe and swift hospital stay.

The Accident

I WAS AT WORK WHEN I received that phone call no one wants to get.

"Your mother has been involved in a car accident," the paramedic said.

As my stomach sank in pain and my hands became sweaty, the voice elaborated, "She was hit pretty hard on the driver's side. A passerby pulled her out of the car because he saw gas leaking."

As my brain desperately tried to focus on the paramedic's words, he described Mom as having no obvious signs of injury or bleeding, but she was walking around somewhat dazed. She also refused to go to the ER. He said he found my number on a piece of paper in the car and asked me what I wanted to do.

I replied, "Take her to the hospital, I am on my way. But wait, sir! Where is my son? She has my six-year-old with her!" He said in a deep monotone voice, "There is no one with her," and hung up.

The Emergency Room

AFTER CONFIRMING JON was at school, it took nearly an hour before I arrived at the small country hospital. I found Mom in a room, way in the back corner of the Emergency department, alone, on a stretcher with one side rail down. She was awake, appeared puzzled about her whereabouts, and even though she knew me, she was not acting normally. She was not concerned about her grandson, the borrowed car she'd been driving, or the other people involved in the accident.

My mom was a recently retired registered nurse and mother of ten. This 74-year-old independent, active person, living on her own and taking zero medications, was suddenly incoherent about her environment. Her confused state was obvious to me. I began to inspect her body, which appeared intact. There was a half dollar size bump and bruise above her right eyebrow and pain when I touched her right hip. She kept lifting her right leg up saying it didn't feel right. There were a couple of skin tears/abrasions, but there appeared to be nothing substantial.

When the ER physician finally came into Mom's room to examine her, I stepped back and watched in silence. As he was leaving, I asked him what he ordered. His response was a chest X-ray, X-rays of her right hip and leg, and some blood work. I casually mentioned the paramedic said she was hit hard on the driver's side, and she was acting confused. I was trying to emphasize that this was not her normal state. I finally muscled up the nerve to ask, "Are you going to order a CT scan of her head?" He did not answer.

It wasn't long before lab personnel arrived and started drawing her blood. The staff member did not identify herself nor did she say what blood work was ordered, so I asked!

Soon afterward, a gentleman entered the room and identified himself as being from Radiology. He checked her armband for identification and asked my mother to confirm her name. He then recited the types of tests ordered and mentioned she would go for a CT scan after the X-rays were taken. This employee followed protocol.

About an hour later I looked up to see two staff members hurriedly pushing Mom's stretcher past her room and down the hall towards the center of the Emergency department. They were taking her to the "Trauma Room" (where only the true emergencies go). I knew this wasn't good.

All at once, several RNs converged on that room with the physician calling out orders. Eventually, one by one, the nurses went back to caring for their patients, leaving the primary RN to monitor Mom while keeping me posted on her progress.

At this point, Mom had two large peripheral IVs, one in each arm, with IV fluids infusing "wide open" (as fast as it could flow). EKG patches were all over her chest and extremities and she was hooked up to a heart monitor and oxygen. There was a urine catheter bag in place, and a bag sitting at the foot of her bed with her cut-up clothes — they'd used scissors to remove them as quickly as possible.

Pain control is always the patient's first concern. Mom was restless and agitated, flopping around in bed. They gave her morphine, which was effective in helping her relax, then sleep.

Finally, the ER physician approached me. He said Mom had sustained a subdural hematoma (bleeding in the brain) which caused her confusion. It was confirmed by the CT scan. She also had several rib and pelvic fractures. Her blood work didn't look bad; mild anemia due to the bleeding. There was no need for a blood transfusion unless the bleeding continued. Due to her head injury, she needed to be transferred to a specialized facility. He said he had already made the arrangements and had spoken to the admitting physician. She was going to be life-flighted to Vanderbilt Trauma Center in Nashville, TN. At this point, it felt like hurry up and wait!

Emergency Room Checklist

❑ Did the staff member identify the department they represent?

❑ Did you hear them say the patient's name and date of birth?

❑ Did you see the staff read the patient's armband and verbally confirm allergies?

❑ Did they say what tests would be performed?

Prior to medications being given:

❑ Did the RN confirm the patient's name and date of birth (by asking aloud and looking at their armband)?

❑ Did the RN say the medication's name and what it is supposed to do?

❑ Did the RN review drug allergies?

Additional things to notice:

- Be sure that the stretcher is in the low position, locked, and the side rails are up.
- Make certain to bring all medications from home.
- Speak up if you question anything.
- Reinforce to your loved one that they will be okay.
- If the patient has an Advance Directive at home, bring it in so a copy may be put in their chart to support their wishes.
- Avoid texting or being on the phone when a staff member enters the room.
- Focus on listening and watching what's going on with your loved one.

The Intensive Care Unit

OURS LATER, MOM ARRIVED at her designated bed inside the trauma ICU after a second CT scan was performed to determine the extent of the bleed in her brain. The neurosurgeon found our family in the waiting room. He explained she was not a candidate for surgery to stop the bleeding. It had to stop on its own or she would die. He elaborated that the second CT scan was not worse than the first which was a good sign, but he would not comment on her prognosis.

It was around 8 p.m. before we were able to see our mom. She lay flat on her back in the same position since arriving at the ER well over 10 hours earlier. She presented pleasantly confused and was cooperating with the nurses. However, it is not unusual for patients to be irritated and uncooperative. (If they are restless and inadvertently exposing themselves, you can get another hospital gown, put their legs into the "arms" of the gown, open in the back. This will cover them.)

I mentioned to the RN that Mom had not eaten all day, and point-blank asked: "Can she get some food?"

After the RN said yes, I then asked if I could help turn Mom off her back, also pointing out she had been lying flat since 10 a.m.

Intensive Care Unit Checklist

Patient's immediate needs vary due to the severity of their condition. Food and water are dependent on their situation.

☐ Ask if they can eat or drink.

☐ What pain control measures are being taken?

☐ Safety measures: are the side rails up?
  Place call light within reach.

☐ Remind patient where the call button is and to not get up without help.

☐ Has the patient been in the same position for many hours? If so, check with the nurse regarding repositioning.

Other considerations:

- Does the patient seem uncharacteristically confused or sleepy?
- Do they experience pain when you touch them? If so, you need to find out why.
- Do they feel extra warm or cold when touched? Is this their normal?
- If the patient feels hot or cold, check to see how many (if any) blankets are on the bed. Make the appropriate adjustments.
- The alarms from the heart monitors and IV pumps are often heard. Do not attempt to turn them off.
- Does the patient want or need anything?
- Dentures and glasses—take them home if not in use.

The Floor

THE NEXT MORNING a third CT scan was done. It showed the bleeding in her brain had stopped!! Mom was more coherent. The neurosurgeon ordered her transfer out of ICU to the Telemetry Unit where they monitor cardiac rhythms (patients wear a small box with wires attached to the chest). This also means a cardiologist gets involved.

So, in addition to the admitting physician, there were now four doctors on Mom's case. The neurosurgeon was no longer involved since surgery was ruled out. A neurologist took over the care for her subdural hematoma. A cardiologist was monitoring her heart because they must have seen some irregularity on the heart monitor (nothing major since no additional tests were ordered). There was also an orthopedic surgeon who evaluated her fractures. He determined no surgery was necessary, they would heal on their own, but he remained on standby.

By the time Mom arrived in her new room, it was near the end of day two. The Foley catheter/urinary bag remained in place and she was still on bedrest. These are the two primary culprits for hospital acquired infections. Normally you want the catheter pulled out as quickly as possible to encourage the patient to get up out of bed as soon as possible. This is key to getting better sooner. The longer we stay in bed, the slower the body will respond.

However, from a nursing point of view, we tend to put off pulling out the catheter. Elderly people require a lot of extra time, especially when it's their first time out of bed. I promised the RN I would stay with Mom and get her to and from the bathroom if the catheter was removed. Bedpans are not an option (except in rare, strict bedrest scenarios). It did take nearly an hour to make that first bathroom trip.

As I helped Mom back into bed for the night, I gave her water and repositioned her to her side. I also pulled the side rails to an upright and locked position placing the nurse's call light within reach. I reminded her where the button was in case she needed help.

"P"

Patient Advocate

THE **PAINFREE** APPROACH begins with **"P"** for Patient Advocate. This is the person who assists, supports, and guides a patient through the healthcare system. Advocates look out for a patient's best interests and help clarify information so the patient may make informed decisions about their health.

Listening, looking, and learning what is transpiring with your loved one are the primary ways of protecting them.

"Teach-back" is a method to clarify one's understanding of the situation. After listening to a nurse or doctor or any staff member, say what they said back to them in your own words. This will help prevent any misunderstandings.

This also works both ways. If you notice a change in the patient, tell the RN. If you question their understanding or lack of urgency, speak up, listen to your gut, and ask the nurse what they think. This will assure comprehension.

P - Patient Advocate Checklist

❑ Listen and watch staff when they enter the room.

❑ Ask questions.

❑ Listen and watch what the patient is doing:
Is their speech clear, are they lying in one spot or moving around?

❑ Is your loved one's behavior outside of their norm?

❑ Tell the RN if you notice a change in their behavior.

❑ Confirm that both the medical providers and the staff members say the patient's full name and date of birth for identification.
(This practice is mandated by the National Patient Safety Guidelines.)

❑ Ask whether any new tests, lab work, or medications have been ordered.

❑ Remember to follow-up on those test results.

❑ Discuss what other departments are involved in your loved one's care; for example, physical therapy, or awaiting a procedure to be done.

❑ Check on their progress; keeping track is helpful.
(See the notes section in the back of this guide.)

❑ Secure your loved one in for the night
(side rails/bed locked/call light).

Time-saving techniques nurses will appreciate:

- Designate one family member to be responsible for making all the calls to the hospital. That one person can then relay the information to the rest of the family. If several people are calling in, the RN has to stop each time, answer the call, and go over the same information again and again. These interruptions mean less time at the bedside.

- Save all requests for the nurse at one time. Items requested often include extra blankets, towels, pillows, water, and pain medication. Make a list. Or if permissible, ask where the closet is so you can help yourself.

- Keep notes to maintain a list of questions or concerns and to help visitors stay informed.

"A"

Ambulate

Now it's time to get moving.

I arrived early the next morning because I wanted Mom out of that bed! Two full days of bed rest doesn't sound like much, but when it comes to the elderly, their system slows down at a greater speed when it's not moving. Lungs, intestines, and blood flow will begin to back up if they don't get circulating.

First things first. Confirm with the RN there are no orders restricting the patient to be on bedrest. All patients can get out of bed unless the physician has written "bedrest." And it is in rare and temporary situations when a patient must stay in bed. For example, if they have blood clots or are having a heart attack. Otherwise, once you know they can get up, then the best time is mealtime!

If a patient is not ready or willing to get to the chair to eat breakfast, then assist them to sit on the side of the bed (versus staying in bed with the head of the bed raised). You can have them hold a pillow across their abdomen for support—it hurts less. Also, you want to remind them to breathe deeply. They may get a little dizzy—it normally subsides quickly. If, after a couple of minutes, they are still dizzy, lay them back down, wait a little while, then repeat.

Once ready to eat, it is better for the patient to cut their own food, open their own milk container, or prepare their own coffee. I know all loved ones want to prepare food on their behalf, but by waiting and watching the patient do the work themselves, it improves their finger dexterity, their hand-eye coordination, and makes them breathe more deeply. This is about the best time to text or use your phone; it allows time for the patient to feed themselves. Of course, help when they struggle to open a bottle or cut food. If you notice, they will get a workout just eating! This is incredibly beneficial to their recovery—it speeds it up.

After any workout, we are tired. A trip to the bathroom after breakfast is always a healthy move. Taking naps is a positive necessity in the healing process.

Feel comfortable calling the nurse for assistance at any time. Families are not replacing the nurse to help the patient to the bathroom; you are the coach. If you do not want to or can't participate, call for assistance. If you are not comfortable doing anything hands-on with the patient, don't. There are plenty of eyes and ears jobs the coach must consider throughout the day.

A - Ambulate Checklist

❑ Sit the patient up on the side of the bed. Allow time for them to get their balance.

❑ If he or she experiences pain with coughing or moving, placing a pillow across their abdomen will help ease their discomfort.

❑ Deep breathing is often helpful with clearing the lungs.

❑ Make sure there is nothing to trip over on the way to the bathroom. IV pumps, electrical cords, and table legs are all potential hazards!

❑ Check that the bed is locked (just lean on it, you will know), and that it is set in its lowest position.

❑ Use a second hospital gown like a robe to conceal the opening in the back.

❑ Put on non-slip socks or shoes before getting out of bed to prevent falls.

❑ When the patient is ready, use a walker, cane, or your arm for support.

❑ For patient safety, move slowly; avoid rushing the patient.

Additional considerations:

- If weak, ask RN for a belt—to be used around their waist (for added support). If worried, have wheel/chair nearby in case patient decides to stop walking.
- Track how many times patient is getting out of bed daily.
- How long are they sitting up in the chair?
- Are they ready to venture into the hallway?
- If they are not getting out of bed, consult with the RN as to why and what can be done to get them moving when it is appropriate.

Ideally, the patient should be in their chair for every meal, tolerating the chair for longer and longer periods of time. Work towards walking in the room, then to the hallway, then down the halls, increasing distance or time (or both). Short frequent walks are more beneficial than one long walk.

Remember that walking (or even, simply getting out of bed):

- Promotes circulation by sending oxygen throughout the body which boosts the healing process, deters infections, and blood clots.
- Expands the lungs preventing pneumonia.
- Improves one's personal outlook (hopefully).

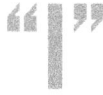

"I"

Infection

HEALTHCARE ASSOCIATED INFECTIONS (HAIs) are infections patients might acquire while they are hospitalized. According to the Centers for Disease Control and Prevention (CDC), on any given day about one in every thirty-one hospital patients has at least one healthcare-associated infection.[11]

Another complication known as hospital-acquired conditions (HACs) are conditions that are not present at the time of admission but may develop while the patient is in the hospital. These include: adverse drug events (allergic reactions or medication errors), falls, blood clots, as well as infections—urinary, central lines, pulmonary, skin, and surgical sites.[12]

Any of these potentially preventable problems or infections lead to longer hospital stays, more medications, more discomfort, and more charges added to the bill.

Good coaching by the patient's advocate will help prevent these complications.

The number one way to prevent the spread of infection is handwashing. This goes for everyone: healthcare workers, visitors, and even the patients! It is recommended to wash with soap and water or rub hand sanitizer for 20 seconds—which is equivalent to singing the happy birthday song twice!

It is difficult and intimidating to say to the staff, doctors, and loved ones: "STOP, wash your hands before you touch the patient." But it must be done if you did not witness the hand washing or the application of antibacterial gel.

Here are a few ideas to help make it easier:

- Just say, "Thank you for washing your hands."
- "Would you mind cleaning your hands before you take the blood pressure?"
- Tape a sign to the foot of the bed (or somewhere visible when entering the room): "Pleaseeee wash your hands!"
- Casually mention, "The sink is over there."
- Alcohol-based hand sanitizers kill most germs so have some nearby. When doctors/staff arrive, squirt some in their hands and smile. (This is my personal favorite!)
- Squirt sanitizer into the patient's hands throughout the day.

Other ways to prevent the spread of infection:

- If visitors are sick (with a mild cough or congestion) ask them to please go home.

- Keep small children at home. Besides dealing with their fears, they can put the elderly at a much higher risk for infection.
- Although housekeeping staff clean the rooms daily, it wouldn't hurt to bring in your own disinfectant wipes to use on the bed rails, the TV remote, the call light, and the bedside table.

Note: Putting on gloves as an alternative to using soap or sanitizer is NOT effective. According to the World Health Organization, "Gloves do not provide complete protection against hand contamination."[13]

This means all doctors, nurses and anyone else coming into physical contact with the patient must either use soap or sanitizer—*then* they can put on their gloves (if necessary).

Note: There are bacterial-induced infections that require/mandate using soap and water prior to touching the patient. Hand sanitizers are not effective in these cases. In this scenario, there will be a sign on the door to let visitors and staff know.

Let's elaborate about preventing infections. There are other considerations besides just washing our hands. It's looking at the whole person/body.

Pneumonia (an infection in the lungs)

Can be due to the position of the body from prolonged bedrest or from not being turned for long periods of time. Can also be due to not raising the head of the bed whenever possible—for example, when they are attached to a breathing machine. (You want the head of the bed up at least 20 degrees.)

Urinary tract infections (infection in the bladder)

Signs of infection include burning or pressure with urination. With the elderly, sudden onset of confusion is frequently seen. It's commonly caused by the extended use of a Foley catheter (urinary bag). Inquire daily when it can be removed—then ensure the patient is getting up out of bed, making their way to the toilet. Using a urinal defeats the benefits of getting out of bed.

Skin break down (caused by continuous pressure on the skin)

This can be due to lying flat on the back. No air can get to the skin (i.e., buttocks) so no blood can move through the skin when it's pressed down. Consider this example: put pressure on your fingernail until it turns white. The reason it turns white is because the blood has been pressed out of the area. Now imagine that happening for days without a break!

Another common area that receives continuous pressure is where the oxygen tubing sits over/around the ears. You'll notice reddened skin, depressed tissue; these are early signs. Or if bone on bone, (i.e., one ankle is on top of the other one) there needs to be a cushion. Place a pillow or folded blanket between knees and ankles. Make sure elbows are not in direct contact with the side rails.

Central line infections (intravenous sites allow IV fluids to flow into the system)

These large bore IV sites (as well as peripheral IV sites) can become infected (you will see a sudden spike in temperature). Either of these infections can cause pain, swelling, redness, or oozing at the insertion site where the IV goes into the vein.

I - Infection Checklist

❏ Did you observe the staff washing their hands or using sanitizer?

❏ If not, ask them to do so OR simply squirt sanitizer into their hands!

❏ Relatives, friends, and children should all do the same before touching the patient.

❏ Look at the patient, are they in the same position as they were four or six hours ago?
If so, turn, reposition to their side, using pillows (or blankets) for support behind their back.
Ask the nurse if you can help them turn your loved one.

❏ Is there an incentive spirometer available?
If not, ask the nurse to get you one (no order is necessary). This is a great apparatus to help expand the lungs. Encourage patients to use it every two to four hours while sitting upright.

❏ Is the urine catheter bag still in place?
Ask the nurse when this can be removed.

❏ When oxygen tubing appears visibly contaminated, ask to replace. Also, look around the ears and face to make sure it's not too tight. It's okay to loosen for comfort.

❏ Look at the IV insertion site. Is there redness, tenderness, or swelling? If so, tell the RN immediately.

❏ If hands, arms or legs are swollen, elevate those limbs on a pillow or a folded towel. Be sure the nurse knows and ask what the swelling means.

"N"

Nutrition

FOODS ARE TYPICALLY REFERRED to as healthy or unhealthy. I categorize foods as those that cause chronic inflammation and those that don't! Chronic inflammation is the culprit for many of the reasons why people are hospitalized. Their bodies become sick because they frequently consume foods that are unhealthy.

These inflammatory foods are the prepackaged, processed, high fat, high sugar foods and drinks that predispose us to chronic conditions that worsen with each passing day unless we change our habits. These conditions or illnesses include diabetes, hypertension, heart disease, stroke, dementia, obesity, arthritis, and even some cancers. Other influencing factors that come into play are inactivity, genetics, alcohol, and tobacco.

So, when we are sick, the body struggles with trying to heal itself. Eating those same inflammatory foods slows down the healing process. On the other hand, making better food choices will help the body heal.

In the hospital, every patient receives a dietary order on the day of admission. These orders vary from nothing by mouth (NPO), to liquids only, full liquids, soft, regular, diabetic, cardiac, and so on. The orders are adjusted (hopefully daily) to the changing needs of the patient.

Please note that those with congestive heart failure are usually on "fluid restriction." It is very important to comply with this restriction and to track daily fluid consumption. Too much water or other liquids can cause the condition of these patients to worsen. It is known as fluid overload. Please consult with the RN regarding maximum amounts of fluid intake.

If you have any questions concerning what a person should and should not have, please consult with your RN. If you would like more information, the RN can set up a meeting with the hospital dietitian; they are a great resource!

Occasionally, diet orders are not written (as in Mom's case). When this happens, the patient does not receive food! Or, another potential error happens when diet orders are not adjusted as the days go by. Discuss this with the RN as well.

Promoting good nutrition will aid in the healing process. For example, Vitamin C foods repair the body's tissue and boost the immune system (among other benefits). Plant-based foods are full of antioxidants and are known to protect or delay cellular damage and lower the risk of chronic diseases.

Basically, what I am suggesting is to choose more fruits and vegetables, eat less meat. Avoid processed, and prepackaged foods. If your loved one prefers meat, steamed or baked chicken or fish are healthier alternatives than fried.

Choose water over soda. Smoothies instead of ice cream. Fruit instead of candy. Soups instead of solids. These choices are better for the body.

You can also Google "Vitamin C foods." Anything the patient likes on that list, bring it in! For my mom, I would bring her an apple a day; sliced it up and left the skin on for added fiber. Although low on the Vitamin C list, it was all she would eat during those first few days plus it helped with constipation. You must be creative and flexible when your loved ones are picky eaters or don't want anything at all. Another thought is the vending machine foods are for the visitors. Avoid giving those prepackaged products to the patient.

N - Nutrition Checklist

❏ Encourage that a piece of fruit is eaten daily.

❏ Suggest water over soda.

❏ Recommend fruit smoothies instead of ice cream.

❏ Avoid red meat (it can cause constipation).

❏ Fiber foods and veggies help best with motility.

❏ Ask if there are any foods the patient should not eat.

"F"

Faith

WHILE IN STRESSFUL SITUATIONS, most people tap into their belief system, higher power, or consult clergy. There are thousands of books documenting the positive effects of faith and the healing connection. Faith in one's recovery strengthens the ability to cope.

With this in mind, I suggest that families and patients tap into their spiritual beliefs for the added support and guidance to get through the trauma. Fostering an optimistic outlook to a person who feels miserable or is discouraged will strengthen their immune system.

An additional approach to assisting with coping mechanisms is to increase the production of endorphins. Endorphins are chemicals that act as opiates, giving us natural pain and stress relief while stimulating our immune system. They circulate in the bloodstream after exercise, but other activities can activate them as well. For example:

- Smiling versus frowning (it requires more muscles to frown, than to smile).
- Humor/laughter. Show your loved one funny videos or pictures they will like. This helps them heal.
- Soothing music.
- Flowers or aromas can induce endorphin production. Be sure to ask the staff about bringing in flowers. Some units (such as the ICU) will not allow them due to the risk of an opportunistic infection from the soil.
- Rubbing their back, shoulders, or feet is usually very comforting.
- Sometimes just sitting quietly in the corner has a calming effect on the patient.
- Depression is a common problem. Encourage patients to play a game on their phone, do word puzzles, or engage them in a card game—whatever they like or used to like. It will distract their negative thoughts.

This brings me to the other side of the bed. Be aware when there is too much activity in the patient's room. Sometimes too many visitors show up at the same time. It becomes a social event, but this can be stressful for the patient. They need rest, and over-stimulation impedes their healing. Taking turns coming in and out of the room may help.

In addition, if disagreements and arguments start, PLEASE take it outside of the room, and down the hall, so your voices can not be heard. Patients don't need the added stress from the kids or extended family members!

Let me end this section with a simple, "Be Nice." Yes, everyone is stressed out, in a hurry, impatient, and wants to be somewhere else.

However, when families add unnecessary tension by being rude to the RN, it hurts all around. Nurses are human too. If an RN gets harassed or bombarded with unrealistic demands every time he or she walks into the room, all this does is make the nurse go into that room as seldom as possible.

Whereas, just introducing yourself and asking the nurse's name can create a more positive tone; a friendly relationship starts. Now the RN wants to come into that specific room as often as possible!

Which is best for the patient?

F - Faith Checklist

❑ Read something inspirational.

❑ Brighten up the room to help the patient smile.

❑ Request that the clergy of choice makes a visit.

❑ Take a stroll to the chapel.

❑ Try to turn the patient's focus to the positive.

❑ Help them to visualize feeling better; offer hope.

❑ Laugh or pray – patient's preference.

The ultimate goal is to turn the patient's focus toward the positive.

For example: if they're complaining about the pain, respond by telling them that means their nerve endings are working! If they say the food tastes bad, respond by telling them that it's a sign of improvement; their taste buds are returning. If they refuse to walk any further, remind them they did better than yesterday. If they complain about the cost of auto repairs (due to an accident), tell them the car did its job because they got to walk away.

"Why worry when you can pray."
Author Unknown

"R"

Remember to Follow-up

WHEN AN RN COMES INTO the patient's room, they have several jobs to complete. Although this is the time to ask all your questions, you must (you WANT to) allow the RN to focus on the immediate tasks—usually it is the medications and the IV fluids hanging on the pump. The medications and numbers must be correct: accurate drug, dosage, and rate. Avoid talking when it is obvious they are reading and adjusting the pump(s). Distractions can definitely lead to errors.

Then, when the RN turns his or her focus to the patient—this is the ideal window to discuss immediate concerns. Yesterday's activities are not so much a factor as the present moment. Sure, you want to follow-up on the tests done yesterday, but you first need to inquire about their present status.

To review the current diagnoses:

Use the teach-back method to gain the clearest understanding of what was just said by the doctor or nurse.

Using this technique is important because this new information is like learning another language. Communication must go back and forth to get the full understanding. You deserve the time it takes to assimilate the information.

Review the meds being given at this time.

Inquire about anything and everything on your mind. For example, pain medication. Do you feel it's helping your loved one? Are they still complaining of pain an hour or two after it was given? Most pain medications should give adequate relief for about 4 to 6 hours. If the medicine is ineffective, discuss it with the nurse.

As coaches, you should become familiar with the medications.

Simplify—make it easy on yourself. Just put in your notes that x drug manages blood pressure every six hours. By learning the names of the meds, why, and when they are administered, you will become aware of any changes, thus preventing a potential error.

Inquire about vitals and tests.

Ask about the most recent blood pressure and heart rate. Also inquire about their oxygen saturation if they are receiving oxygen. Remember to ask about their lab results, x-rays, or procedures, as well as any pertinent information, for example, blood sugars or heart rhythm. Make notes.

R - Remember to Follow-up Checklist

❑ Are there any additional conditions being treated?

❑ What are the results of tests: X-rays, MRI, CT, etc.?

❑ What are the lab results? What do they indicate?

❑ What was the outcome of the procedure?

❑ Have any new medications been prescribed? What side effects are possible?

❑ How are the patient's vital signs? Blood pressure, heart rate, oxygenation?

❑ If on a heart monitor, how is his or her heart rhythm? Regular, irregular, fast, slow, or perfect?

❑ Make a list of questions or concerns.

❑ Confirm your understanding of what is explained to you by repeating it back in your own words.

❑ Remember to put your phone down when someone walks into the room so you may give your undivided attention.

Remember Medications Checklist

☐ Did the nurse confirm the patient's name, date of birth, and drug allergies before administering medication?

☐ What condition does the medicine treat?

☐ Become familiar with the names of the medications and the times they are given. They are generally ordered every 6, 8, or 12 hours.

☐ Keeping a list will help prevent a wrong or duplicate medication being given (med error).

☐ Is the pain medication helping? It should bring some relief. If not, discuss it.

☐ Are there any side effects?

☐ Is the medicine working to help the problem?

☐ If constipation is an issue, ask about a stool softener.

☐ Do not take medications from home unless authorized.

☐ Speak up if you have any questions or concerns.

Doctors. Have you seen any lately?

It's hit or miss with doctors. Ask the nurse if they know the time frame the MD might be making his or her rounds. If you continue to miss them, call their office, ask to schedule a time to speak directly to the physician or to the nurse practitioner/physician assistant. Have your list ready.

If the primary is the hospitalist, then there is no office to call. In this scenario, leave a note taped to the front of the chart asking the doctor to call or to leave a number where he or she can be reached.

At the end of every shift the RN gives the summary report to the oncoming RN. The report is either given at the bedside or at the nurse's station. If the nurses (or doctors) are discussing the patient at the bedside, join in and listen. You are part of the healthcare team.

"E"

Eliminate

WE ALL DO IT, so we must discuss it.

Urine output is generally measured. But it's temporary. Once patients are eating and drinking and are without kidney or cardiac issues, then measurement is no longer necessary. When in doubt, confirm with the nurse.

In the meantime, there is a plastic "hat" in the toilet for the women and a urinal for the men that make measurement easy. The nursing staff will empty them, no worries. There is also usually a piece of paper taped to the wall in the bathroom to allow staff quick and easy documentation of I & Os—intake and output. It is customary to track how much goes in, the percentage of food eaten, and the amount of fluid consumed. In other words, the intake. If it is being tracked, you want to help keep it up to date.

The other area of concern is when there is too much coming out or none at all. The nurse needs to know if patients are having a problem with either constipation or diarrhea so appropriate medicine can be ordered to resolve the situation. Vomiting and sweating are additional ways the body eliminates. The nurse needs to know if the patient is suddenly sweaty or is nauseated.

"E"

Educate

As a patient advocate, you want to learn as much as you can about your loved one's medical conditions, associated tests being ordered, and the general workflow within the hospital. This awareness puts you in a position to prevent mistakes and mishaps. For example, a staff member may enter the wrong patient's room or has the wrong chart in hand. An alert observer can help avoid a potential error.

Being cognizant of the medications' names will also heighten your ability to notice when there is a change. Speak up when you question something; ask for clarification. Listen.

By figuring out the terminology and understanding the pros and cons of the treatment plan, you are better able to explain the situation to the patient so they can make an informed decision about their own health and healthcare.

This is especially important for the elderly. They may or may not want to undergo all forms of medical treatment/regimens. They know they are closer to the end than the rest of us. Quality of life might be more important than having surgery to stay alive an extra few months.

The term "foreseeable outcome" means predicting the consequences of an action. There may be occasions when one must question the benefits of a procedure or surgery. There are circumstances when doctors offer surgical procedures in an effort to try anything to extend the patient's life.

The question is: Do the advantages outweigh the disadvantages? Recovering from surgery is difficult considering the extra pain and other side effects. Is it worth it? What is best for the patient? Sometimes, it's okay to say no, but thank you.

Years ago, I was working in the Intensive Care Unit. A cardiac surgeon recommended surgery on an 86-year-old diabetic patient in my care. Using medical jargon, he explained his rationale for the operation to the woman's daughter.

When he was done, there was a pause. So, I spoke up. I summarized the physician's words in layman's terms. I explained that basically, if the patient had this surgery, it would not lengthen her life or change her current status. I made it clear that her mother would most likely endure a long and painful recovery. And that was IF she recovered, due to her uncontrolled diabetes and her deteriorated state of mind and body.

I recall the surgeon giving me a disapproving look, but I knew it was the right thing to do. As an advocate for the patient it was my job to fully inform the family. Not to mention, I would be signing the consent as a witness, acknowledging that the pre- and post-procedures were explained and understood.

The daughter chose for her mom to have the surgery.

About two or three months later, I was at work. The daughter approached me as a stretcher carrying her mom was being whisked down the hall. She said, "I wish I would have listened to you." Her mother made it through the surgery that day, but it had been a downhill battle ever since.

The daughter continued by saying, "Just now, she is returning from having her third surgery, removing her remaining leg." So now her mom was a bilateral above-the-knees amputee; the side effects of the surgery and diabetes.

My mom had made it clear to me and the rest of my siblings, she wanted nothing to do with extending her life. She made herself a DNR (Do Not Resuscitate) years before the accident and reminded me of this during her hospitalization.

If the patient is of clear mind, they should be encouraged to decide what medical treatment they want to undergo. Of course, if they are not of clear mind, then the families and caregivers should carry out their wishes as documented in the patient's advance directives.

Patient-centered care is a triangular model where all healthcare providers, family members, and caregivers work together, collaborating as a team in the best interests of the patient. It addresses the patient with a holistic view: their physical needs, emotional well-being, and spiritual beliefs. It also involves active engagement by the patient to improve overall satisfaction and outcome.

E – Educate Checklist

❑ Learn about the medical conditions.

❑ Learn about the medications.

❑ Learn about the hospital flow; who is doing what for your loved one.

❑ Encourage your patient to move.

❑ Encourage good food choices.

❑ Make the patient smile and deep breathe.

❑ Watch for changes/abnormal behavior.

Overall, always remember to:

Engage

- When patients and their families are active participants in their healthcare, both their personal
  and economic outcomes improve. There was a
  time when patients entered the hospital and no
  one asked any questions or participated—that was
  the expectation. Times have changed. It is now all
  about patient-centered care. All involved take an
  active role in the recovery. Everyone benefits!

Exercise

- Move extremities even if they can't move on their
  own. For example, a stroke patient can lose one side
  of his body. Some ideas to prevent contractures: put
  a small ball in the palm of the hand, move the fingers and move the forearm, then the whole arm/
  leg. Watch how the physical therapist works with
  the patient and copy it. Walk with them as often
  as you can, increasing frequency and or duration.
  This gets blood flowing to all the organs, supports
  the healing process, prevents constipation, and improves their general outlook.

Check for Edema

- If fingers are swollen, remove rings, and take them
  home. Ring cutters are available (you may have to

check with the ER to borrow one). If arms or feet are swollen, elevate them on pillows. Notice daily if swelling is improving or worsening. Always discuss with the nurse.

Prevent Falls

- Is the bed locked and in its lowest position? Are electrical cords out of the path to the bathroom or the chair? Are IV pumps and other equipment out of the way? Make certain your loved one always wears non-slip shoes/slippers. Does the patient need an assistive device such as a cane or a walker for added support? They do help to improve balance. The RN can arrange the necessary equipment.
- Are side rails up after patient gets back into bed?

Use Incentive Spirometers

- These are disposable instruments that help the lungs expand. A member of the respiratory department or the nurse can deliver one. It's best to use it every two hours while awake and sitting up. All patients benefit from using incentive spirometers. They help prevent pneumonia.

Discharge Instructions

Finally, it's time for the Super Bowl! The patient (quarterback) gets to go home! Your RN will review the discharge orders which include the summary of why the patient was admitted, any additional diagnoses, medications to be taken, diet, activity level, and the list of physicians with whom to make follow-up appointments.

Additional agencies such as home health or physical therapy may be ordered as well. You then sign off acknowledging the instructions and home you go. Understand that the patient may still be in pain and even dazed by the events of the preceding days.

You need to follow these same **PAINFREE Guidelines** at home:

"P" Patient advocate: Patient or family caregiver should ask questions for clarification.

- Use the teach-back method at time of discharge to make sure you understand what to do and how to do it.
- Confirm the foods or activities that should be avoided.

- Verify that hospital records will be forwarded to the patient's primary physician.
- Medications often change upon discharge from what was taken prior to admission. Be sure you have a clear understanding of the new meds, what to take and not take. Compare and confirm the names and dosages from the list you have at home.

"A" Ambulate: Increase walking duration and/or frequency.

- Track daily how far or how often they walk.
- Use assistive devices (i.e., cane, walker).
- Keep walkways free of objects.
- Remove rugs to prevent falls.

"I" Infection: Wash your hands three or more times daily to prevent infection.

- Follow the discharge orders for dressing changes and showering directions.
- Avoid touching areas where sutures are present.
- Signs of infection: increased pain, swelling, redness, oozing at the incision site.
- Additional signs are fever for no apparent reason, or any worsening symptom (i.e., cough).
- Notify the doctor's office if there are signs of infection.

"N" Nutrition: Eat foods that will enhance the healing process.

- Follow diet orders.
- Indulge in Vitamin C-rich foods.

- Consume water, lean meats, and low sodium products.
- Avoid processed, sugary foods.

"F" Faith or Fun: Try to smile and laugh.

- Seek out spiritual support of choice.
- Keep the faith. There's always hope.
- Encourage social interaction.

"R" Remember: Don't forget these other details.

- Ask about all test results; try to get copies.
- Coordination of care—are those agencies visiting the home as scheduled?
- Have they delivered all necessary equipment? If not, speak to the RN in charge of your case.
- Do you have all the supplies you need (i.e., blood sugar device, bandages, etc.)?
- Pain is a part of recuperating. The more the patient moves, the faster the pain will lessen with each passing day. The narcotics are a temporary solution.

"E" Eliminate: Is the plumbing working properly?

- Constipation is a common problem. Take the stool softener as ordered, avoid red meat, drink water, eat fruits, fiber, vegetables, and walk. This will get the intestines moving.
- When was the last bowel movement?
- If there are any problems with urination, diarrhea or constipation, call your doctor or hospital discharge nurse for guidance.

"E" Educate: Learn everything you can about their medical condition(s).

- This understanding helps keep symptoms under control.
- Know what medications treat which conditions.
- Know the best time of day to take the medications.
- Be aware of medication side effects.
- Know what to do in case of emergency.

The bottom line is to be an active participant to promote recovery. Continue their use of the incentive spirometer for at least an extra week or two following discharge. Make certain they take medications as directed and keep the follow-up appointments with the physician(s).

If you have questions or concerns, call Virtual Healing at **727-729-2099** or email **Maureen@virtualhealing.com** for assistance.

Conclusion

THE HUSTLE AND BUSTLE OF our lives, along with the need to answer an influx of texts, emails, and phone calls, as well as the added distractions of social media, videos, and podcasts can make most of us feel a bit overwhelmed.

Then the phone rings. Someone you love is in the hospital. Your stress level quadruples. When you turn to Google to learn about their condition, you end up reading material on the high numbers of preventable hospital complications caused by healthcare errors.

As you continue your research you will find that hospitals are woefully understaffed. This leads to increased work pressure for doctors, nurses, and aides. It in turn increases the chances of those medical errors and the likelihood that a medical professional will simply miss important changes in a patient's condition.

Evidence-based data suggests patient-centered care will expedite recovery both during and after hospitalization. The registered nurse is the primary link between patients, families, and the rest of the hospital staff including doctors and all the departments. But with the nursing shortage, patient centered care is difficult to achieve. The nurses are caring for more patients, while physicians and specialists are writing more orders, and families and friends expect more information about their loved one's illness.

There is good news. Research indicates that when families, friends, or caregivers participate in the patient's care, the number of healthcare errors are reduced, and patient outcomes are improved.

Even better, the healthcare industry acknowledges the importance of a patient's circle of support and is actively encouraging them to become part of the healthcare team, thus, emphasizing patient-centered care.

Still, many people are hesitant to take an active role in a loved one's recovery. They don't feel qualified to participate, especially when the hospital's own staff are trained—and paid—to provide proper care.

What these caring families need to understand is that mistakes *do* happen, even when understaffing and overwork are not the contributing factors. In many cases it is simply the human factor, something technology cannot alter (yet). That's why having an extra pair of eyes to see something abnormal and an extra pair of hands to help with the power of touch will provide an undeniable benefit in enabling patients to recover without complications.

Yes, it is the registered nurse's job to oversee all aspects of patient care. The task is daunting:

- Performing and documenting physical exams
- Administering medications

- Changing surgical dressings
- Monitoring vital signs and overall conditions
- Supervising reactions to procedures and medications
- Implementing many individualized physician orders
- Interpreting and following-up with their results
- Providing education to both the patient and their families

… in addition to responding to the unforeseen issues that occur along the way.

The reality is this. Taking an active role in helping your loved one during their hospitalization increases the odds of them having a safe and swift experience.

This is where the **PAINFREE Guidelines** come in. They are a handy reference to help families and caregivers encourage recovery and stay alert to subtle changes that may indicate the start of a relapse. It helps you think about all the different aspects necessary to promote recuperation and prevent mishaps.

Don't be sidetracked when a patient balks (and they will) at your determination to get him or her up and moving. Recovery is hard and uncomfortable, and even really painful at times. But the goal *is* recovery with return to normal activities.

You need to be resolute in your efforts as a proactive member of the healthcare team!

Patient Centered Care

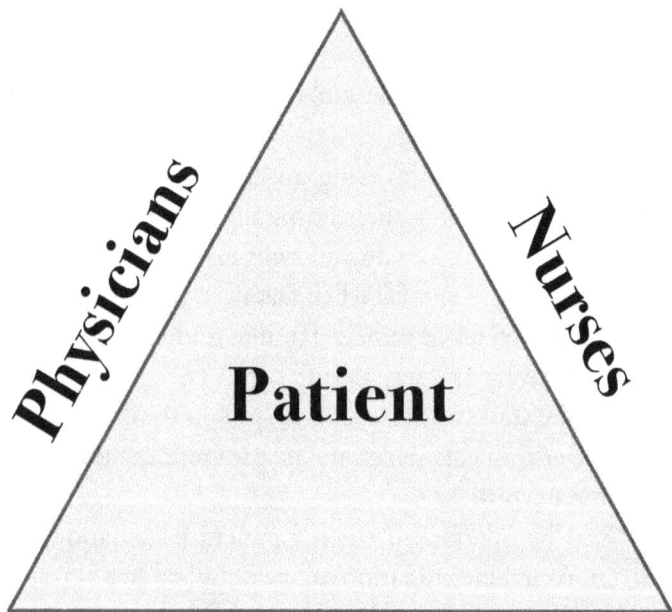

Physicians

Nurses

Patient

Families, Caregivers

Glossary

Advance Directives

Legal documents that allow you to spell out your decisions about end of life care ahead of time. It is a legal way for your family caregivers, friends, and healthcare professionals to carry out your wishes.

Advocate

One who assists, supports, and guides a patient through the healthcare system.

Ambulate

To walk, move about.

Anemia

Hemoglobin or red blood cells are low. There are three main causes: blood loss, lack of red blood cell production, or high rate of red blood cell destruction.

Bed Rest

Physicians will prescribe this for patients whose medical condition may worsen if the patient gets out of bed. If it is not written as an order, patients are encouraged to get up as often as possible.

Bedside

Bedside nursing implies doing hands-on nursing care.

Blood Clot

Also known as a venous thromboembolism, this clot forms in the deep veins of the legs, arms, or pelvis. They develop from being sedentary, especially after surgery.

Blood Sugar/Blood Glucose

This is the main sugar found in your blood. It comes from the food we eat and then the blood carries it to all the body's cells to use for energy.

Central Line

A long tube (catheter) that goes into a vein. It ends up in the heart or empties into a large vein near the heart.

Chronic Inflammation

The body responds to an infection, then the infection goes away, but the body remains in a long-term state of inflammation resulting in chronic health problems.

CT Scan

Computed tomography (CT) is a type of imaging. It uses special X-ray equipment to make cross-sectional pictures of your body. These scans assist doctors to identify internal bleeding, fractures, blood clots, and other conditions.

Do Not Resuscitate (DNR)

This is a legal document that expresses a patient's wishes not to be kept alive by artificial means.

Edema

Swelling caused by injury, inflammation, medications, pregnancy, or infections.

Electrocardiogram (EKG)

A test that records the electrical activity of the heart. Patches are applied to connect the wires for the reading. It is common for staff to leave the patches attached to the body, however they can and should be removed.

Family Members

Includes friends and caregivers; anyone who wants the best for the patient.

Foley Urine Catheter

A urinary catheter is a tube placed to drain and collect urine from the bladder.

Fracture

A break in a bone.

Incentive Spirometers

Disposable devices or instruments that help lungs to expand and helps to prevent pneumonia.

Interdepartmental

Involving or existing between two or more departments such as:

Dietary—Supplies all nutritional support.
Laboratory—Blood is analyzed under a microscope; areas include microbiology, hematology, chemistry,

and blood banking. Other specialty testing and analysis may be performed.

Environmental Services (Janitorial)—Front line team who disinfects, sanitizes, and cleans the hospital rooms and floors keeping a healthy environment for all.

Radiology—Science dealing with X-rays (photographing organs, bones, etc.); may include several specialty testing and procedures.

MRI

Magnetic resonance imaging uses a large magnet and radio waves to look at organs and structures inside your body. These tests are used to examine and diagnose a variety of conditions.

Nurse

Includes Registered Nurses (RN) who have a two- or four-year nursing degree. Licensed Practical Nurses (LPN) have a one-year degree and may give oral medications. In some states LPN's are referred to as Licensed Vocational Nurses (LVN). And, Certified Nursing Assistants (CNA) help patients perform basic daily tasks.

Peripheral IV

A peripheral intravenous line is a small, short, plastic tube, known as a catheter. It is put into a vein, usually in the hand or arm, to allow healthcare professionals to infuse fluids and/or medications.

Skin Tear/Abrasion

A scraped area in the skin; a superficial cut.

Subdural Hematoma

A collection of blood between the outer covering and the surface of the brain.

Telemetry

This continuous cardiac monitoring allows the cardiac waveforms to be transmitted to nearby nursing units so they may read and interpret heart rhythms. Patients wear (or carry) a "box" attached to wires on the chest.

Trauma ICU

An Intensive Care Unit equipped to provide specialized care to trauma patients who suffer from serious injury.

Vital Signs

Assessment of blood pressure, heart rate, respiratory rate, and temperature. "Pain level" has been added as the fifth vital sign.

X-rays

Type of radiation called electromagnetic waves; these images create pictures of the inside of the body.

References

1. Sipherd, Ray. "The third-leading cause of death in US most doctors don't want you to know about" Modern Medicine, Published 02/22/2018, Updated 02/28/2018; https://www.cnbc.com/2018/02/22/medical-errors-third-leading-cause-of-death-in-america.html

2. Rodziewicz, T. & Hipskind, J. "Medical Error Prevention" National Center for Biotechnology Information, U.S. National Library of Medicine, 8600 Rockville Pike, Bethesda MD, 20894 USA, 05/05/2019; https://www.ncbi.nlm.nih.gov/books/NBK499956/

3. Bureau of Labor Statistics, U.S. Department of Labor, Occupational Outlook Handbook, Registered Nurses; https://www.bls.gov/ooh/healthcare/registerednurses.html (visited October 31, 2019).

4. Rosseter, Robert. "Nursing Faculty Shortage" American Association of Colleges of Nursing, April 2019; https://www.aacnnursing.org/News-Information/Fact-Sheets/Nursing-FacultyShortage

5. Rosseter, Robert. "Nursing Faculty Shortage" American Association of Colleges of Nursing, April 2019; https://www.aacnnursing.org/News-Information/Fact-Sheets/Nursing-FacultyShortage

6. Needleman, J., Buerhous, P., Stewart, M., Zelevinsky, K., & Mattke, S. "Nurse Staffing in Hospitals: Is There A Business Case for Quality?" Health Tracking, Agency for Healthcare

Research and Quality, U.S. Department of Health and Human Services, Published 01/25/2006, Updated 01/25/2007; https://psnet.ahrq.gov/issue/nurse-staffing-hospitals-there-business-case-quality

7.   Rosseter, Robert. "Nursing Faculty Shortage" American Association of Colleges of Nursing, April 2019; https://www.aacnnursing.org/News-Information/Fact-Sheets/Nursing-FacultyShortage

8.   Bureau of Labor Statistics, U.S. Department of Labor, Occupational Outlook Handbook, Registered Nurses, https://www.bls.gov/ooh/healthcare/registerednurses.html (visited October 31, 2019).

9.   Gaugler, J. Ph.D., James, B. Ph.D., Johnson, T. Ph.D., Marin, A. Ph.D., and Weuve, J. M.P.H., Sc.D., "Alzheimer's Disease Facts and Figures, 2018" Alzheimer's Association, Chicago, IL; Alzheimer's Association. 2018 Alzheimer's Disease Facts and Figures. Alzheimer's Dementia 2018; 14(3):367-429; https://www.alz.org/media/homeoffice/facts%20and%20figures/facts-and-figures.pdf

10. Duncan, G. W. (2013, November 4). Historical Foundation of Universal Healthcare. Retrieved from https://www.selffundingmagazine.com/article/historical-foundation-of-universal-healthcare.html

11. HAI Data. (2018, October 5). Retrieved from https://www.cdc.gov/hai/data/index.html

12. AHRQ Tools To Reduce Hospital-Acquired Conditions/ Agency for Healthcare Research and Quality, 2016; https://www.ahrq.gov/hai/hac/tools.html

13. "Glove Use Information Leaflet—Patient Safety" World Health Organization. Updated August 2009; https://www.who.int/gpsc/5may/Glove_Use_Information_Leaflet.pdf

About the Author

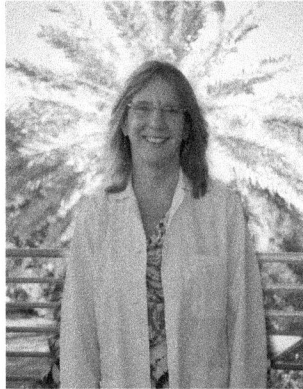

MAUREEN "MIMI" HEALY is a family nurse practitioner who initially worked as a registered nurse in emergency rooms, intensive care units, and other hospital specialty areas for over twenty-five years. Incorporating patients and their families to be active participants of the healthcare team has always been an integral part of her nursing.

Maureen's advocacy for patient safety and engagement embraces the growing trend to empower patients to take more control over their health. She promotes and encourages patients and families to make healthier lifestyle choices while continuing to treat both acute and chronic conditions.

As an independent healthcare educator with Virtual Healing, Inc., a service Maureen created to provide on-line and phone-based support to people managing their health needs at home. The company serves as a resource for patients as well as their caregivers to expedite hospital recovery using a holistic approach.

In her spare time, Mimi pursues her love of sports by playing on a co-ed softball team and golfing whenever possible. She is a member of the Woodlawn Hitting Club, an avid bicycle rider, and continues to adjust enthusiastically to her new roles as author and entrepreneur.

Acknowledgements

I want to thank my son, Jon Camacho for his ever-present support and belief in me and this endeavor.

My siblings: Mike, Mark, Kathy, Dan, Paul, John, Ray, Joe, and Steven for their endless love. My nephew, Karl Healy, PharmD, MS, BCPS, BCCCP for his uniquely detailed views.

My friends for sharing the journey with me in making this book a reality: Daisy Jabas, RN, CPRS; Allison Moore; Beverly Clark; Eileen Kosey; Kysa Smith, CPA; Sue Ross, RN; Robert F. Camacho, CPA; Maurice Bransford, RN; Michele Bratcher, RN; and Mayra and John Schmidt.

And to

All my former patients who unknowingly participated in strengthening my skills so I may continue to help others.

Thank you from the bottom of my heart!

Notes